ARRHYTHMIA AND PALPITATIONS:

When You Have No Clue and Your Doctor Can't Find What's Wrong!

Krystie Love

This book is from the What'z the Occasion "Quick Guide Series". The "Quick Guide Series" take complex issues and explains them in an easy to read, comprehend, and follow format. Each book in the "Quick Guide Series" is sixty pages or fewer. No more fumbling through hundreds of pages to find answers.

Contents

Disclaimer

This information is not presented by a healthcare provider and is for educational and informational purposes only. This book is not a substitute for medical advice. All medical advice should come from your healthcare provider. Do not substitute the advice in this book for a diagnosis or treatment you have received from a healthcare provider. This book is based on my opinion on the subject. I am not a physician. You should always, check with your healthcare provider first with questions about your health. Do not disregard professional advice you have received from your healthcare provider nor should you ever delay your care due to you reading or hearing something.

If you have not already, it is important to first get evaluated by your healthcare provider to rule out a more serious health condition. Your healthcare provider can perform various tests to determine your particular health condition. You can then speak with your healthcare provider about possible solutions found in this book to help address your health concerns.

Additionally, there are several supplements recommended in this book; therefore, it is important to speak with your healthcare provider before taking any supplements to ensure you are taking the right combination, dosage, and if these supplements are appropriate for your particular health condition as some supplements may interfere with medication or lead to health related issues.

INTRODUCTION

Palpitations feel like a flutter in your chest. Your heart may feel like it is racing or beating entirely too fast, or a feeling of missing beats. Palpitations may leave a fluttery feeling that may be felt in the chest area. You may experience hard rapid beats that can be felt in the throat, neck, and or chest area.

In the middle of the night, you may awake with your heart beating at 150 BPM or faster. Scared, you rush to the emergency room only to be told your vital signs are normal and there is nothing wrong with your heart. Then you are sent home still scared, frustrated, with no real solutions, except you did learn a few new words such as tachycardia, arrhythmia, palpitations, atrial fibrillation, and a few others.

This book is designed to help you identify a few causes of heart palpitations to get relief. This book is intended to be short, concise, and to the point to avoid wordiness. I also suffered from palpitations and all I wanted was the facts; instead, I found long drawn out articles, books, and videos that ended up frustrating me just trying to find answers to questions.

When I suffered from palpitations, I was discouraged hearing stories of people who had suffered for years and could not find relief. To be honest, I thought living a normal life was in the past. I went back and forth to the emergency room over a dozen times and saw several specialists and still, no one had the answer. Then, I started talking with people to find different ways they overcame their heart palpitations. There were just so many causes of heart palpitations that it became overwhelming.

Running back and forth to the doctor, not one time did my doctor mention other causes such as helicobacter pylori. There are many causes as to why you may be experiencing your heart acting differently. Sometimes physicians do not have all the answers and it seems all too often they want to blame anxiety on a problem you know is real. This book will allow you to talk with your physician and explore different known causes of palpitations to find what works for you.

As with many of us who suffer from palpitations, we have spent countless amounts of time and money only to be told that there is nothing wrong with our heart. Still, we find ourselves running back to the emergency room only to be referred to our primary care physician, who does not have a clue.

You have seen a cardiologist on numerous occasions and had almost every heart related test available. You had a stress test and worn a heart harness; still no one can help, not your physician, not your cardiologist, not even your friends. In fact, your physician and or cardiologist may have prescribed you beta blockers or even calcium channel blockers, which alone may cause other conditions; thus, making your condition even worse.

I truly hope that there is a solution for you in this book. I can relate. Remember, I too suffered from palpitations; however, I overcame my palpitations. I took everything I found as I researched this subject and compiled all my findings that have worked for me and others just like US.

ARRHYTHMIA

Heart issues affect people worldwide. An adult's heart beats in the range of sixty to one hundred beats per minute (BPM) at rest.[8] "If your heart beats faster than one hundred beats per minute or less than sixty BPM you may have arrhythmia";[8] however, in a person who is athletic, "A lower heart rate at rest implies more efficient heart function and better cardiovascular fitness. For example, a well-trained athlete might have a normal resting heart rate closer to 40 beats a minute".[8] Just because a person has a heart beating under sixty BPM, that does not necessarily indicate a heart condition.

There are two major types of Arrhythmia, Tachycardia, and Bradycardia.

Tachycardia is when the heart beats at a fast rate of more than one hundred BPM.

Supraventricular (SVT): One of the most common arrhythmia. The heart is beating so fast it cannot fill with blood before it contracts. SVT may cause issues with the top chamber's AV nodes, and atria. The heart may beat as fast as 200 BPM.

Ventricular tachycardia (V-tach or VT): A serious form of tachycardia. Ventricular tachycardia occurs when the heart beats fast and at an irregular rhythm. This occurs due to the ventricles squeezing chaotically. When this happens, the heart is not pumping an efficient amount of blood to the body and lungs. Oftentimes, the person will need immediate medical attention to prevent brain damage or even death. Ventricular tachycardia may signal an underlying heart condition.

Signs of tachycardia include:

- ✓ Fainting, near fainting
- ✓ A flutter that you can feel in the chest
- ✓ Breathlessness (dyspnea)
- ✓ Dizziness
- ✓ Chest pain
- ✓ Lightheadedness suddenly feeling weak

Bradycardia is when the heart beats at a slow rate of less than sixty BPM.

Bradycardia: This commonly affects the elderly. Some causes of bradycardia are when sinus nodes that transmit electrical impulses do not fire properly or transmit at a slower rate. Tissues may block the sinus node before they reach ventricles and the atria. This can cause the heart to beat slowly. Other causes such as age, medications, and heart disease all can play a factor.

Signs of bradycardia include:

- ✓ Heart palpitations
- ✓ Angina (chest pain)
- ✓ Shortness of breath
- ✓ Problems concentrating
- ✓ Confusion
- ✓ Exercising difficulties

- ✓ Dizziness/ Fatigue
- ✓ Lightheadedness
- ✓ Fainting or feeling like fainting
- ✓ Sweating

Some other examples of arrhythmia:

Atrial Fibrillation (AFib): AFib is an abnormal pattern. This happens when the right and left atria which make up the upper heart chambers are contracting irregularly. This in return causes the heart to beat at a faster rate. The atrial chamber may cause the heart to quiver, flutter, or even contract. This can cause blood clots in the atrium which can cause clotting in the brain; thus, leading to a stroke. AFib is the most common arrhythmia. It is estimated that 33.5 million people worldwide suffer from AFib.[17]

Symptoms of Atrial Fibrillation:

- ✓ Palpitations
- ✓ Fainting, feel like fainting
- ✓ Angina (chest pain)
- ✓ Breathlessness
- ✓ Weakness
- ✓ Dizziness

Atrial flutter: Atrial flutter is a form of supraventricular where the heart randomly quivers in the atrium. The heart beats fast, but in a normal rhythm. Without treatment, this condition may lead to atrial fibrillation. Some people who have atrial flutter will commonly experience a heartbeat of 250 to 350 BPM.

Symptoms of Atrial Fibrillation:

- ✓ Palpitations
- ✓ Fast steady pulse
- ✓ Shortness of breath
- ✓ Finding it hard to exercise
- ✓ Finding it hard to perform daily activities
- ✓ Chest discomfort
- ✓ Tightness in chest
- ✓ Dizziness
- ✓ Lightheadedness
- ✓ Fainting
- ✓ Feel like fainting

People who are at a higher risk of developing atrial fibrillation may have some of these risk factors listed below:

- ✓ Heart failure
- ✓ Previously had a heart attack
- ✓ Acquired/ Congenital valve abnormalities
- ✓ Diabetes
- ✓ Acute illness
- ✓ High blood pressure
- ✓ Recent upper chamber surgery
- ✓ Thyroid dysfunction
- ✓ Alcoholism (binge drinking high risk)
- ✓ Chronic lung disease

Wolff-Parkinson-White Syndrome: A person with Wolff-Parkinson-White Syndrome has an extra connection in their heart at birth. This extra connection (accessory pathway) enables electrical signal to go around the atrioventricular node. By doing this, the signal moves from the atria to the ventricles early and are transmitted abnormally back to the atria. This can lead to a fast heartbeat, experiencing heart palpitations, dizziness, and even fainting.

Sinus Tachycardia: Your heart is beating normal; it is just beating at a fast rate.

There are several other factors that can affect the way your heart functions.

- ✓ Alcohol
- ✓ Drugs
- ✓ Diabetes
- ✓ Heart disease
- ✓ Hypertension
- ✓ Hyperthyroidism
- ✓ Stress
- ✓ Scarring of the heart (One way this can occur is after a heart attack)
- ✓ Smoking
- ✓ Herbal treatments
- ✓ Supplements
- ✓ Health related conditions
- ✓ Medications
- ✓ Structural change (heart)

ELECTROLYTES

Electrolytes primary function is to "regulate nerve and muscle function, hydrate the body, balance blood acidity and pressure, and help rebuild damaged tissue".[8] It is essential that the body has a well-balanced level of electrolytes to ensure the body runs efficiently. The body is dependent upon electrolytes. A balance of electrolytes is essential in keeping people alive.

Some major electrolytes include:

Potassium: An imbalance may lead to hyperkalemia and hypokalemia

- Hyperkalemia: Too much potassium in the body
- Hypokalemia: Not enough potassium in the body
- Potassium can be found in fresh fruit and vegetables

Calcium: An imbalance may lead to hypercalcemia and hypocalcemia

- Hypercalcemia: Not enough calcium in the bloodstream
- Hypocalcemia: Too much calcium in the blood
- Calcium can be found in green leafy vegetables, yogurt, and milk

Sodium: An imbalance may lead to hypernatremia and hyponatremia

- Hypernatremia: Too much sodium in the body
- Hyponatremia: Not enough sodium in the body
- Sodium can be found in salt

Chloride: An imbalance may lead to hyperchloremia and hypochloremia

- Hyperchloremia: Too much chloride in the body
- Hypochloremia: Not enough chloride in the body
- Chloride can be found in salt

Magnesium: An imbalance may lead to hypermagnesemia and hypomagnesemia

- Hypermagnesemia: Too much magnesium in the body
- Hypomagnesemia: Not enough magnesium in the body
- Magnesium, can be found in green leafy vegetables, bananas, lentils, and nuts

Phosphate An imbalance may lead to hyperphosphatemia or hypophosphatemia

- Hyperphosphatemia: Too much phosphate level in the body
- Hypophosphatemia: Not enough phosphate in the body
- Phosphate can be found in meats, poultry, nuts, and fish

If there is an imbalance in electrolytes then the person may experience serious health issues such as:

- ✓ Arrhythmia
- ✓ Weakness
- ✓ Seizures
- ✓ Blood pressure issues, and other health conditions
- ✓ Coma
- ✓ Cardiac arrest
- ✓ Irregular heartbeat
- ✓ Fast heart rate
- ✓ Fatigue
- ✓ Constipation
- ✓ Lethargy
- ✓ Seizures
- ✓ Nausea
- ✓ Vomiting
- ✓ Diarrhea
- ✓ Abdominal pains
- ✓ Weakness in muscles
- ✓ Muscle cramping
- ✓ Irritability
- ✓ Confusion
- ✓ Headaches
- ✓ Numbness
- ✓ Tingling

Magnesium

Magnesium is vital in maintaining a healthy lifestyle. Magnesium deficiency may lead to weakness in your muscles, irritability, and yes, irregular heartbeats. Our bodies need and depend upon magnesium to support over 300 biochemical reactions that are within our bodies.[12] When the body is deficient in magnesium, our bodies do not function normally. Magnesium is essential in controlling the body's nerve and muscle function.

Magnesium plays a major role in regulating the heart rhythm. A low level of magnesium may put a person at risk for an irregular heartbeat and or heart palpitations.[2] In addition; magnesium deficiency can cause spasms that create severe chest pain which can lead to another heart condition known as angina.

Did you know that about eighty percent of people are deficient in magnesium?

Below are magnesium rich foods:

- ✓ Seeds
- ✓ Nuts
- ✓ Whole grains
- ✓ Beans
- ✓ Leafy green vegetables

To get a better understanding of magnesium, and the role it plays on the heart I recommend that you view a video (http://www.spring.org.uk/the1sttranspor) on YouTube by Dr. Sanjay Gupta a cardiologist from York. In the video, Dr. Gupta discusses a study about the benefits of magnesium as it relates to palpitations. Dr. Gupta also recommends a magnesium supplement to use for palpitation relief. Dr. Gupta is one of only a few of cardiologists that recommend or talk about using magnesium as a treatment for heart rhythm issues.

Symptoms of magnesium deficiency:

- ✓ Muscle twitches
- ✓ Osteoporosis
- ✓ Mental disorders
- ✓ Muscle cramps
- ✓ Fatigue
- ✓ Muscle feel weak
- ✓ High blood pressure
- ✓ Asthma
- ✓ Irregular heartbeat

Magnesium Blood Test

Although you had your magnesium level tested by your physician, it may leave you with false hope of accuracy, and here's why.

When there is a low level of magnesium, the body will take magnesium from cells to keep the blood level at a normal range. Oftentimes, physicians rely on a traditional blood test to check for magnesium deficiencies. In fact, it is estimated that up to ninety percent of magnesium deficiencies go undetected by the use of traditional blood test.[6] The numbers are startling; however, physicians still continue to base patients' magnesium levels on traditional blood tests.[6]

A more accurate blood test that is used to measure magnesium levels is the RBC test. The RBC is designed to test red blood cells in the blood stream. This test is more accurate than when a physician uses a traditional blood test.

Other test used to check magnesium levels:

- ✓ EXA Test
- ✓ Ionic
- ✓ Serum
- ✓ Loading/Tolerance test

Request A Test is a company that you can personally request a magnesium test without a prescription from your physician (in most states). Request A Test (http://requestatest.com/) is located throughout the United States and specializes in low cost testing. The process is simple. You enter your zip code, pay a nominal fee, and go to the nearest facility for testing.

Calcium

Calcium is the most abundant mineral in the body; therefore, having a deficiency in calcium can have a drastic impact on the heart. Calcium is essential for vascular contraction, and widening of blood vessels. In fact, calcium plays a key role in controlling blood pressure. In addition to other areas such as hormonal secretion, muscle function, and nerve transmission. Low calcium levels can lead to an abnormal heartbeat.

On the other hand, a person can have heart issues by having an excess amount of calcium in the body. By using calcium supplements and not balancing the levels with an adequate amount of vitamin D, this can lead to heart related conditions such as palpitations. This can cause an excess of calcium in the heart's muscle tissues; thus, possibly causing a high heart rate. Vitamin D is needed to help absorb the excessive calcium that may be settling in other areas besides the bones.

For this reason, experts recommend that a person get calcium from foods as opposed to using supplements. Some excellent sources of calcium are foods such as beans, and fat free Greek yogurt. For example, Greek yogurt has almost 450 mm of calcium along with other recommended daily vitamins such as vitamin D.

Some great sources of calcium include:

- ✓ Sardines and salmon
- ✓ Spinach and kale
- ✓ Legumes and beans

- ✓ Soy milk
- ✓ Almond
- ✓ Rhubarb
- ✓ Sesame seed
- ✓ Orange juice
- ✓ Broccoli
- ✓ Cheese
- ✓ Whey protein

Vitamin D

Vitamin D is important for the body not just because it protects our teeth and helps to prevent osteoporosis; however, Vitamin D is also important for heart health. In fact, Vitamin D is vital in maintaining a healthy cardiovascular system. Many people associate vitamin D with sun exposure and dairy products. When a person goes outside, the sun produces a sufficient amount of vitamin D; however, that is not always the case. For example, people with darker skin or a woman in perimenopause may not take in an adequate amount of sunlight as they may not be absorbing the sunrays as in previous years

Furthermore, suntan lotions can play a role in the absorption of vitamin D. Today it is recommended that suntan lotion be used to protect the skin from dangerous sunrays. In addition, diet, age, and health, are other contributing factors that can play a role in vitamin D deficiency. When a person is deficient in Vitamin D, there is a higher risk for "heart attacks, congestive heart failure, peripheral arterial disease (PAD), strokes, and the conditions associated with cardiovascular diseases, such as high blood pressure and diabetes".[13] Vitamin D helps to ensure that magnesium and calcium are regulated throughout the body. Vitamin D is responsible for regulating over 200 genes in the body.

Calcium which can be found in foods such as dairy, broccoli, and fish all need vitamin D to be absorbed and distributed throughout the body. When vitamin D levels are low, the person may experience palpitations and abnormal heart rhythms.

As with calcium, vitamin D also plays a key role in the absorption of magnesium. Low vitamin D affects the overall levels of magnesium. Low levels of magnesium can lead to palpitations, abnormal heart rhythms, muscles spasms, anxiety, and more.

Taking vitamin D supplements can affect the body negatively. When a person consumes too much of vitamin D from supplements, it can affect the heart. The extra vitamin D in the system raises calcium levels in the blood.

This extra absorption of calcium that the body is taking in can cause symptoms such as:

- ✓ Constipation
- ✓ Digestive issues
- ✓ Loss of bone density
- ✓ Kidney stones
- ✓ Muscle pain
- ✓ Increase risk for a heart attack
- ✓ Increase risk for a stroke

Thiamine Deficiency

Thiamine is also known as B1. Thiamine deficiency as it relates to heart palpitation is controversial. At one time, thiamine was looked at as an alcoholic's disease. In the U.S., a manifestation of thiamine deficiency is the Wernicke-Korsakoff syndrome. This syndrome is often found in chronic alcoholics who have poor eating habits; however, anyone or people who use drugs, gastrointestinal disorders, and have HIV/AIDS also can develop this deficiency.

Today the link between thiamine deficiency and the heart is becoming more apparent. Thiamine plays a vital role in heart health. Thiamine is responsible for our nervous system, muscle functions, digestive system, and carbohydrate metabolism. Due to the body not producing thiamine, it is necessary for us to get the thiamine from other sources such as foods and or supplements.

Foods that are rich in thiamine include:

- ✓ Whole grain bread
- ✓ Meat
- ✓ Fish
- ✓ Legumes
- ✓ Whole grains
- ✓ Cereals, read the breakfast cereal box to locate brands that are rich in thiamine
- ✓ Nuts
- ✓ Dairy products
- ✓ Oranges
- ✓ Beans
- ✓ Seeds

- ✓ Vegetables such as beets, Brussel sprouts, asparagus, and acorn squash

There are two types of thiamine deficiencies: wet beriberi and dry beriberi.

Wet beriberi is related to the heart and circulatory system.

Some symptoms associated with wet beriberi include:

- ✓ Tachycardia/Palpitations
- ✓ Widening of blood vessels
- ✓ Heart failure
- ✓ Enlarge heart
- ✓ Edema
- ✓ Retention of salt
- ✓ Retention of water
- ✓ Malaise
- ✓ Anorexia
- ✓ Shortness of breath
- ✓ Waking up short of breath

Dry beriberi is associated with nerves. This can reduce muscle strength.

Some dry beriberi symptoms include:

- ✓ Loss of appetite
- ✓ Muscle cramps (calves)
- ✓ Pins and needles (lower extremities)
- ✓ Paralysis
- ✓ Mental symptoms
- ✓ Enlarged heart

- ✓ Muscle function/paralysis
- ✓ Pain
- ✓ Vomiting
- ✓ Issues with speaking
- ✓ Involuntary eye movement

Countries that have access to foods that contain thiamine have a much smaller chance of developing beriberi. With that being said, there have been cases reported is some pregnant women who had severe morning sickness (hyperemesis gravidarum) during pregnancy. Additionally, it has been seen in a person after they have undergone bariatric surgery.

Potassium

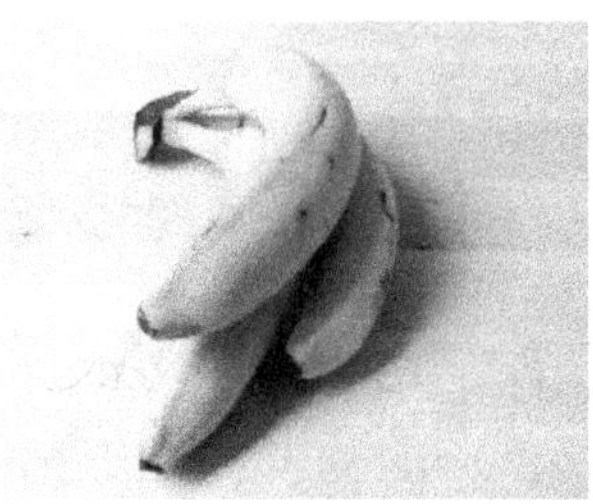

Potassium is an electrolyte that plays a vital role in the body's health. Potassium helps in regulating the water balance between body fluids and cells. Maintaining the recommended amount of potassium helps to maintain a normal heart rhythm by regulating muscles and heart nerves. Potassium is tricky in that too much potassium can have a drastic impact on the body just as not enough potassium. An unbalanced level of potassium can cause irregular heartbeats, such as a slow or fast beating heart or even death.

If the potassium level is too low (hypokalemia), the heart will not function properly. The heart could beat too slow, or too fast. The heart may just beat erratic. If the potassium level is too high (hyperkalemia), then again the heart could suffer; thus, causing arrhythmia.

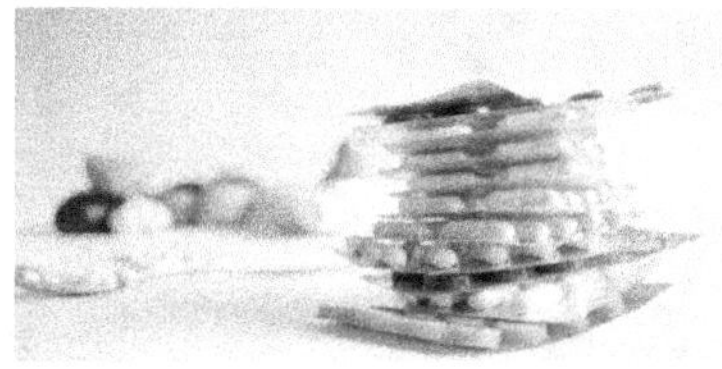

When thinking about taking a potassium supplement, it is recommended that you speak with your physician. Your physician can test your potassium level to determine if a problem exists. When taking potassium supplements, it is recommended that you do so only under your physician's supervision.

When we think of potassium, a banana seems to come to mind; however, there are a lot of other foods that are rich in potassium. A few of these foods are listed below.

- ❖ White potato: A white potato has about 900 mg of potassium
- ❖ Sweet potato: A sweet potato has about 900 mg of potassium
- ❖ Beets: One cup of beets has between 400-500 mg of potassium
- ❖ Canned black beans: Canned black beans have between 700-800 mg of potassium
- ❖ White beans: White beans contain over 1000 mg of potassium.
- ❖ Plain white yogurt: Plain white yogurt contains over 550 mg of potassium
- ❖ Canned salmon: Canned salmon has over 450 mg of potassium
- ❖ Banana: A banana contains over 400 mg of potassium
- ❖ Avocado: An avocado has over 700 mg of potassium

As stated above, it is not recommended that you take a potassium supplement or any other supplement unless directed by your physician. As you can see there are a lot of foods that contain potassium.

Aloe

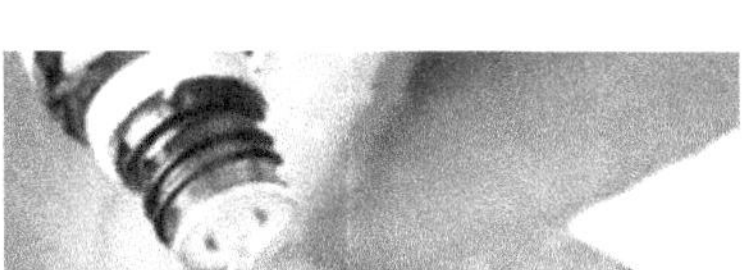

Aloe (consumption) is another supplement that may offer relief. Many people who have taken aloe gel and juice had experienced relief from their palpitations. The benefit of aloe dates back to the 18th and 19th centuries. Aloe is a thick gel that comes out of an aloe leaf. Aloe gel consists of ninety-seven percent water, glycoproteins, and polysaccharides.

In fact, aloe vera juice is abundant in vitamins. Aloe vera juice contains "vitamins A, C, D, E, and a combination of B vitamins: B1, B2, B6, B12, folic acid, and niacin. Aloe also contains such minerals as copper, magnesium, calcium, potassium, zinc, sodium, and iron as well as amino acids and enzymes".[1] By consuming aloe juice this helps to regulate and strengthen arteries and veins. Additionally, aloe vera is rich in nutrients which "help to dilate the capillaries and boost blood oxygenation, thereby offering therapeutic benefits on the cardiovascular system".[1]

There was a study that followed 5,000 people over a five-year period who was taking aloe vera and psyllium fiber. The study showed a decrease in angina attacks. Participants' cholesterol, blood sugar and triglycerides had also decreased. Additionally, eighty-five percent of participants' heart rhythm was normal. Of the 5000 participants, 2,151 who had high blood pressure, taking beta blockers, or calcium channel blockers, or diuretic medications used to treat hypertension and angina showed improvement. The participants' medication was reduced to half of what they were previously taking. [1]

Some experts recommend using aloe to relieve palpitations; however, on the flip side some experts recommend not using aloe vera. Just as some people have successfully cured palpitation with aloe, some people had reported that by drinking aloe on a daily basis they developed palpitations; therefore, aloe could be a double edge sword. One study revealed that people who are taking aloe vera may contribute their palpitations to the supplement. The study followed 514 participants who were having some kind of side effect from aloe vera.

Of the 514 participants in the study, 53.33% of women and 46.67% of men had reported that they developed palpitations as a side effect from aloe vera.[2] Today there are many products that contain aloe vera; therefore, reading labels is important. For example, some toothpaste and medications contains aloe vera. Aloe gel is used in toothpaste due to the ability to fight cavities. Some people may have palpitations from aloe, by eliminating the aloe hidden in products you are using may help to alleviate your palpitations.

Did you know that there is aloe in some products we use every day?

- ✓ Aloe has been approved by the FDA to be used as flavoring
- ✓ Aloe is used as a natural antioxidant
- ✓ Aloe can be found in cosmetics
- ✓ Aloe is also found in food supplements.
- ✓ Aloe is used to treat constipation

THE NATURAL CHANGE

Androgen

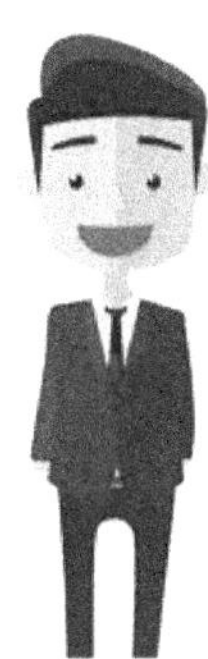

I started with androgen as it may be shocking and unbelievable to some people that men go through a natural transition similar to menopause. Men go through androgen which is somewhat a male version of menopause. This transition is just like a woman's except androgen is more gradual than that of women.

When men reach about forty they start to have a decline of about one percent each year in their testosterone. A young man may have a testosterone level that exceeds 1000 nanograms per deciliter. Compare that to an older man in his eighties. An older man in his eighties may have a testosterone level of about 200 per deciliter; however, some men in their eighties may still have a normal level of testosterone.

Below are a few symptoms of androgen:

- ✓ Palpitations
- ✓ Cardiovascular
- ✓ Anxiety
- ✓ Low sex drive
- ✓ Hot flashes
- ✓ Erection dysfunction
- ✓ Osteoporosis

During androgen the testosterone level drops as the autonomic system fluctuates. Although, research is still being conducted, some clinical findings have indicated that low levels of testosterone may increase the risk factors for cardiovascular disease. Some men may experience palpitations and night sweats. This is caused by an overactive autonomic system. When a man's autonomic system becomes overactive it can cause a drop in testosterone which can lead to palpitations.

Below is a list of activities that can accelerate the change:

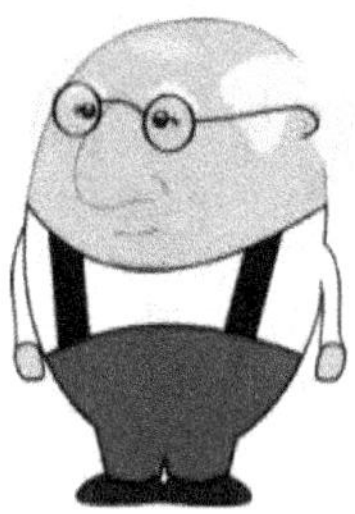

- ✓ A large amount of weight in the abdominal area
- ✓ Being overweight such as obese
- ✓ Stress
- ✓ Illness

- ✓ Tobacco
- ✓ Drugs
- ✓ Alcohol
- ✓ Mental illness
- ✓ Disease
- ✓ Less sexual activity

Today there are remedies available for men to help relieve androgen symptoms. Some ways to combat symptoms and or lower risk include making lifestyle changes. This may include incorporating regular exercise, maintain a healthy diet, eliminate caffeine, antidepressant, add supplements, or take androgen replacement therapy.

If you are thinking about taking androgen replacement therapy, there are a few risks that you should be aware of. Some risks include developing or worsening prostate cancer and heart disease, to name a few. Before deciding on using androgen replacement therapy:

- ✓ Analyze your symptoms
- ✓ Consider current health
- ✓ Consider family history
- ✓ Consider current and previous lifestyle (all healthy and unhealthy behavior)
- ✓ Speak with your physician about the pros and cons

Female Menopause

When we think of menopause we traditionally think of missed periods. We may also link menopause to hot and cold flashes; however, there are several other symptoms that can be associated with menopause. One common symptom of menopause that is barely mentioned is heart palpitations. Some women may experience heart

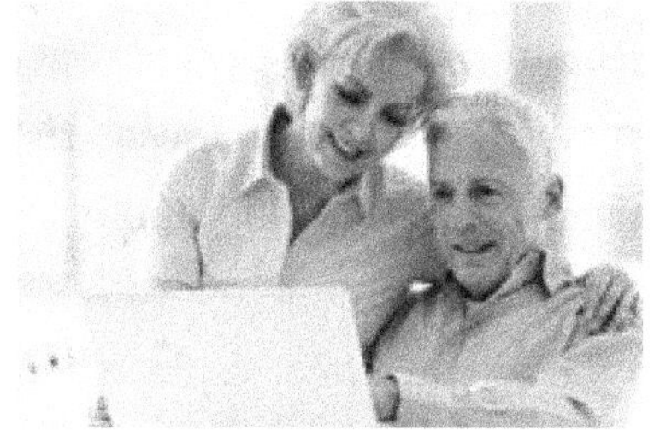

palpitations during perimenopause and menopause. Unfortunately, women can experience menopause symptoms for years before perimenopause to years after menopause.

As hormones (estrogen and progesterone) fluctuate, this in return can lead to overstimulation of the heart. This overstimulation causes a fluctuation in hormones which causes issues with the rhythm of the heart. The imbalance of hormones

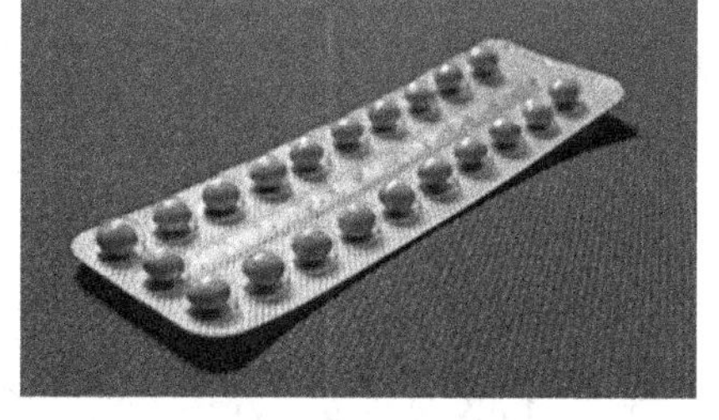

plays a significant role on the heart, which puts women at higher risk for heart disease after menopause.

Some women seek relief from palpitations through hormone replacement therapy (HRT). This should be discussed with your physician who can perform the needed test and properly evaluate your situation to decide if HRT or another alternative is best for you.

Hormone replacement therapy does have some risks involved. Some studies show that if taken early enough in the transition, HRT may prevent heart disease. However, some studies show that there are risks regarding HRT and should only be taken when it is necessary. These studies have shown a higher risk for a woman to have a stroke, blood clots in legs, cancer, or heart disease.

A few interesting facts:

Women are at a lower risk for a heart attack (before menopause), then men.

Women are at a higher risk for a heart attack (after menopause), then men.

When it comes to the survival rate of heart attacks, men have a higher survival rate then women.

A few Signs of Female Menopause

- ✓ Palpitations, fast heartbeat
- ✓ Chest pains
- ✓ Shortness of breath
- ✓ Dizziness
- ✓ Hot flashes
- ✓ Cold flashes
- ✓ Night sweats
- ✓ Weight gain
- ✓ Irregular periods
- ✓ Genetics
- ✓ Chemo/radiation
- ✓ Removal of ovaries
- ✓ Drugs
- ✓ Diet
- ✓ Lifestyle

Helicobacter Pylori

Helicobacter pylori (H. pylori) is a bacteria that is linked to gaseous issues. H. Pylori can cause inflammation and ulcers in the stomach and the duodenum. A person can contract H. pylori from people, contaminated food, and or water.

One interesting fact about H. pylori is that majority of people who have this infection does not have symptoms. Some experts believe this is because the person may have been born with a resistance to fight the infection.

Below are some symptoms associated with H. pylori:

- ✓ Pains in abdomen such as an ache and or burning sensation
- ✓ Pain in the abdomen that tends to worsen when the stomach is empty
- ✓ Fast heart rate
- ✓ Weight loss
- ✓ Burping
- ✓ Nausea
- ✓ Loss of appetite
- ✓ Bloating

One study revealed that people with a heart condition such as atrial fibrillation were twenty times more likely to test positive for H. pylori.[7] A person, who has tested positive for H. pylori, is more likely that their C reactive protein (CRP) is five times higher than normal.[7] The CRP is a substance that a person's liver produces due to inflammation. When a high level is present, it indicates inflammation.

Although there are more studies that need to be conducted on H.

pylori and heart rhythms, the link to the heart may be the autoantibodies the person is infected with. Under normal circumstances, the autoantibodies attack acid pumps located in gaseous cells; however, the autoantibodies may attack different pumps such as cardiac cells which can lead to arrhythmia.

Hiatus Hernia

A hiatus hernia or hiatal herma is when a portion of the stomach protrudes into the chest. The esophagus is the pipe where the food goes down. The esophagus pushes itself through the muscular wall which painfully separates the abdomen and the chest cavity. A person who suffers from a hiatus hernia may experience palpitations.

Palpitations may occur if the vagus nerve becomes irritated. The person may have symptoms such as shortness of breath and acid reflux. The shortness of breath occurs by how the hernia is impacted by the diaphragm. A hiatus hernia is most common in a person who is obese or over the age of fifty.

Below are a few other symptoms associated with Hiatus hernia:

- ✓ May experience heartburn
- ✓ The person may have black stools
- ✓ Regurgitation of food/liquids back into the mouth
- ✓ Acid reflux
- ✓ Difficult when trying to swallow
- ✓ Chest pain
- ✓ Abdominal pain
- ✓ Vomiting blood
- ✓ Passing blood

To be diagnosed for a hiatus hernia; your physician may request an upper endoscopy, or a barium swallow. A barium swallow is when a person drinks a special solution and undergoes a special x-ray to allow the physician to view the esophagus. Endoscopy is when an endoscope (flexible tube) is placed down the throat to allow the physician to view the esophagus, duodenum, and stomach.

Gastrocardiac Syndrome

Gastrocardiac syndrome is also referred to as Roemheld syndrome. Gastrocardiac syndrome is when "A person may experience an extremely low or high heart rate during or after they eat... This is from stomach acids that cause reflux".[4] Oftentimes, the person may find some relief once the person begins to burp.

There are two types of triggers associated with gastrocardiac syndrome, mechanical and neurological. The mechanical triggers *"...occur when pressure is placed on the fundus of the stomach or the esophagus. When the increased epigastric pressure occurs the diaphragm's position is elevated and puts pressure on the heart and vagus nerve. Hiatal hernias are known to be a significant mechanical trigger of Roemheld syndrome"*.[4]

A neurological trigger occurs when there is an increase in the vagus nerve pressure which affects performance. *"When the vagus nerve is compressed your heart rate and blood pressure decrease and in doing so the body's autonomic nervous system is triggered creating a catecholamine dump into the bloodstream. The increased circulating catecholamines cause a massive increase in blood pressure and heart rate"*.[4]

The symptoms may be more severe after a large meal or due to overeating. Eating is not the only trigger associated with the gastrocardiac syndrome. Gastrocardiac syndrome can be triggered by sleep or strenuous activities when pressure is applied to the abdomen.

The three types of gastrocardiac syndrome:

❖ **Dystonic:** False angina accompanied by sweating, irritability, and sleep disorder

❖ **Kardialgichesky:** Pain in the heart due to physical exertion, accompanied with shortness of breath, and palpitations. Triglycerides are much higher than in other gastrocardiac syndromes.

❖ **Arrhythmic:** Systolic and diastolic pressure

Below are a few other symptoms associated with gastrocardiac Syndrome

- ✓ The person may experience hot flashes
- ✓ Some form of arrhythmia
- ✓ GERD
- ✓ Sinus bradycardia that progresses to sinus tachycardia
- ✓ Hypotension that progresses to hypertension
- ✓ The person may experience silent reflux (no symptoms)
- ✓ May feel like everything is spinning (vertigo)
- ✓ PVC's
- ✓ Anxiety
- ✓ Angina
- ✓ Trouble with breathing
- ✓ Trouble sleeping (insomnia)
- ✓ Syncope
- ✓ Tired to weakness and or fatigue
- ✓ Ringing in the ears (tinnitus)
- ✓ Heart condition such as atrial fibrillation (AFib)

- ✓ Frequent coughing
- ✓ A person may clear their throat constantly
- ✓ Heart disease
- ✓ Sudden cardiac death

Heartburn/GERD

Acid reflux has been known to affect millions of people. Acid reflux is when the lower esophageal sphincter doesn't close properly or opens too frequently. This opening allows acids from the stomach to move up the esophagus. When the acids move up the esophagus, you may experience burning which is identified as heartburn. One of the most common causes of acid reflux is a hiatus hernia.

Acid reflux fall under two types.

The first type is heartburn reflux (gastro-esophageal reflux disease). Gastro-esophageal reflux disease (GERD) is when the person experiences symptoms such as heartburn, clearing of throat, hoarseness, a feeling of a lump in the throat, and chronic coughing.

The second type of acid reflux is throatburn reflux (laryngopharyngeal reflux). Throatburn reflux (LPR) is when the person does not have symptoms of heartburn.

The heartburn associated with acid reflux can be felt in the lower esophagus which is in the same area as the heart. When this happens, there is a chance that acid reflux can cause heart palpitations and chest pains. The esophagus can bring on ectopic beats; thus, causing palpitations.

Symptoms associated with acid reflux oftentimes mimic different heart conditions. That is why it is always important to speak with your physician first and use this book as a reference with your physician to get to the root cause of your heart issues.

Some causes and symptoms of Acid Reflux:

- ✓ Eating a large meal and then lying down can worsen symptoms
- ✓ Eating the going to bed , even a snack
- ✓ Obese and overweight
- ✓ Smoking
- ✓ Hiatus hernia
- ✓ Pregnant: Increase in hormones and pressure from the fetus, often goes away after birth of the baby
- ✓ Obese or overweight
- ✓ Citrus and spicy foods
- ✓ Fatty foods
- ✓ Foods containing tomato
- ✓ Mint
- ✓ Carbonated drinks
- ✓ Both tea and coffee (caffeinated and decaffeinated)
- ✓ Medications: Some medications such as aspirin, muscle relaxers, blood pressure medications, and beta blockers

DIET PLAYS AN IMPORTANT FACTOR

Diet

Diet can play a major role in heart health. Foods that contain processed sugar, high in carbohydrates, and sodium can cause heart palpitations. Additionally, eating rich and spicy foods can trigger heartburn which could cause palpitations.

Crash or fad diets that promote rapid weight loss can deprive the body of the necessary nutrients needed for the body to function properly. Depriving the body can cause the body to lack nutrients needed daily, cause dehydration, and weaken the immune system. This in return can cause stress on the body including the heart which can lead to irregular heartbeats. For example, water plays a key role in heart health. A dehydrated heart can lead to palpitations; therefore, it is important to drink the daily recommended water.

Below is a list of other possible causes for palpitations

- ✓ Dietary supplements
- ✓ Caffeine
- ✓ Alcohol
- ✓ Drugs
- ✓ Soda/pop

If you are having heart palpitations, then you may need to stop drinking caffeine. Caffeine is one of the major causes of heart palpitations. It is important to stop drinking teas, pop, sugar, and artificial sweeteners. Artificial sweeteners have been shown to cause palpitations.[5]

Energy drinks are loaded with caffeine because it speeds up the heart. Some energy drink contains 120-200 mg of caffeine while others contain even more, 300-500 mg caffeine. [7]

Some brands of energy drinks may be a little deceptive about listing everything on their product label. For example, "The consumer group tested 27 popular energy drinks. Eleven didn't list the amount of caffeine on the label. Among the 16 products that did, five had more than 20% more caffeine than the label claimed. One had about 70% less".[7]

The recommended daily amount of caffeine is about 400 milligrams for a healthy adult. This is cut in half for a pregnant woman, who is allowed about 200 milligrams of caffeine daily.

Monosodium Glutamate

Monosodium glutamate (MSG) is a food enhancer that may be causing your heart palpitations. MSG is found in processed and canned food. MSG is also commonly found in Chinese foods. There is controversy among experts concerning MSG. Some research indicates a link between palpitations and MSG, while others do not. The FDA has acknowledged that some people may just have an allergic reaction to MSG.[16]

Some symptoms that have been reported include:

- ✓ Headache
- ✓ Flushing
- ✓ Sweating
- ✓ Facial pressure or tightness
- ✓ Numbness
- ✓ Tingling
- ✓ Burning
- ✓ Sensation
- ✓ Heart palpitations
- ✓ Chest pains

SOME COMMON CAUSES OF PALPITATIONS

Dental Hygiene

Yes, poor dental hygiene can cause heart issues.

It is recommended that you visit your dentist on a regular basis. By not brushing and flossing your teeth daily, bacteria can form in your mouth which can lead to inflammation. This inflammation can turn into a disease called gingivitis. Untreated, gingivitis can cause periodontitis or periodontal disease.

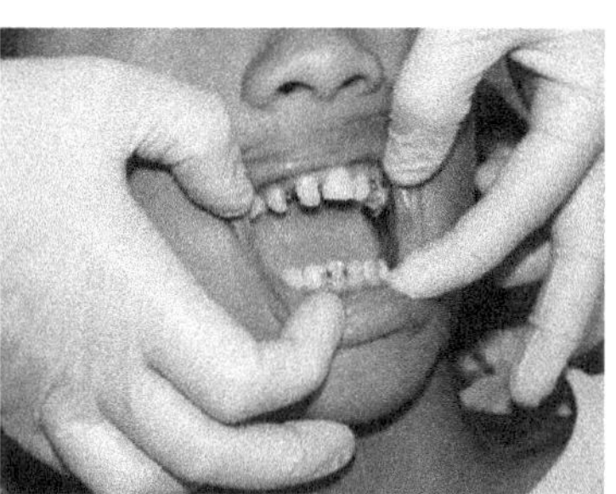

Once periodontitis or periodontal disease sets in, this can cause the gums to become red, sore, bleed, and separate from the teeth.

When the teeth separate from the gums, bacteria can then enter the bloodstream.

The bloodstream may allow the bacteria to travel to the heart's arteries.

Then, it can begin to harden and cause a disease known as atherosclerosis, which can cause heart disease.

Urinary Tract Infection (UTI)

Yes, a urinary tract infection (UTI) can lead to heart palpitations. Although it is more common for women to have a UTI, it is possible for men to have one as well. It is probable that a woman will have at least one UTI in her life. It is probable that majority of men will never have a UTI.

The bacteria from a UTI in a woman can move to the uterus; thus, spreading the infection to the kidneys. From there, the infection can move into the blood stream. It is important for you to treat the condition immediately.

Some symptoms of a UTI:

- ✓ Rapid heart rate
- ✓ Rapid breathing
- ✓ Fever
- ✓ Tremors
- ✓ Frequent urination
- ✓ A feeling of still having to urinate after your done
- ✓ Blood in urine
- ✓ Organ failure

Postural orthostatic tachycardia syndrome (POTS)

Postural orthostatic tachycardia syndrome (POTS) is when a person stands up, and their heart rate increases by thirty or even forty beats

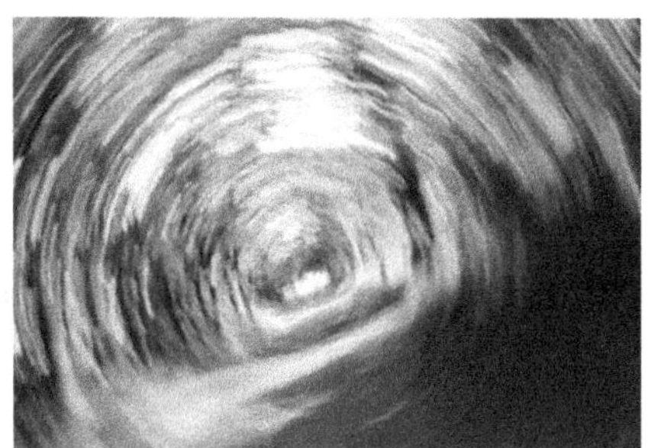

per minute (BPM). Or within five- to -thirty minutes of standing up the person finds their heart beating 120 BPM or faster. The person may experience a sudden drop in their blood pressure; begin feeling dizzy, and or faint.

This condition occurs due to the person's heart not getting enough blood when the person stands up (orthostatic intolerance). To compensate for the lack of blood, the heart will beat more rapid to improve blood circulation.

Some people with POTS experience other issues upon standing. When the person stands up, their legs, and or feet may become a deep purplish or a reddish color; however, upon sitting or lying back down, their legs oftentimes return to normal. This is due to blood pooling in their blood vessels. Some people with POTS had reported pooling in their lower extremities all the time.

POTS can affect anyone regardless of their age or sex; although, POTS mainly affects women. It is not known as to what causes POTS. However, it is believed that it occurs after the person has had trauma, major surgery, or a viral illness. This is just a brief summary of POTS. People with POTS are faced with several symptoms such as brain fog, chronic pain, and digestive issues, to name a small few. Millions of people around the world have POTS and have to live with these symptoms and more.

Listed below are a few symptoms associated with POTS:

- Lightheadedness, dizziness
- Heart palpitations
- Shortness of breath
- Blurred vision
- Chronic pain
- Fainting
- Headache
- Brain Fog
- Tiredness
- Gastrointestinal symptoms
- Head, neck, or chest discomfort
- Fatigue
- Sleep disorders
- Difficulty exercising
- Anxiety
- Coldness or pain in the extremities

If you think you may have POTS, then you should speak with your physician and or cardiologist.

POTS, is a misunderstood syndrome and not all healthcare providers know how to treat people with POTS. Be sure you find a good healthcare provider who knows how to treat people with POTS.

ILLEGAL AND LEGAL DRUGS AND THE HEART

Legal Drugs

Some over the counter medication are linked to fast heart rates. For example, one side effect of aspirin is a fast heartbeat and both Tylenol and aspirin list breathing issues as a side effect.

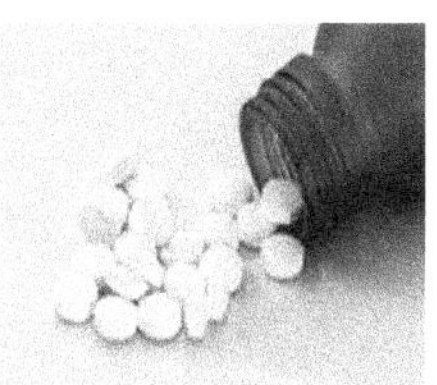

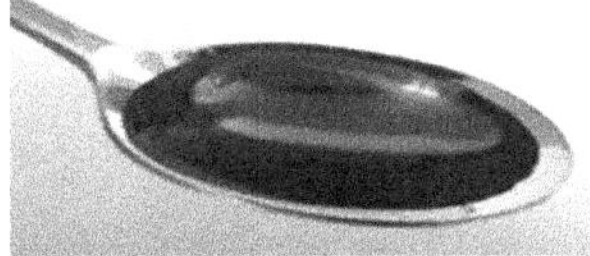

Have a cold? Many cold medications in your medicine cabinet have ingredients in them that can cause a fast heartbeat.

If you are on medication, it is recommended that you research the side effects of your medication. Speak with your physician about your symptoms, to determine if your medication is related to your heart issue.

Be careful when adding supplements to your diet. Many supplements are not regulated by the FDA. Some are made in other countries that have little regulations.

If you decide to use supplements, make sure you buy them from a reputable company.

Some medications that can cause a fast heart rate

- Some asthma inhalers
- Antibiotics
- Antidepressants

Illegal Drugs

Many people think that cannabis mellows them out and makes them chill. Smoking cannabis can make your heart rate increase. There are over one hundred types of cannabinoids in cannabis. We mainly know about the most prevalent types of cannabinoids which are tetrahydrocannabinol, known as (THC) and cannabidiol, known as (CBD).

THC is a drug that can cause anxiety and psychosis. Some people report being paranoid after smoking cannabis. THC can expand blood vessels, which in return speeds up the heart. Illegal drugs are dangerous and should be stopped immediately. If you are using illegal drugs, seek help immediately. Illegal drugs can cause all sorts of health issues or even death.

There are many types of street drugs which each can affect the heart differently. If you already have a heart condition, using street drugs can worsen your condition. Street drugs can slow or speed up the heart, cause a heart attack or some other heart failure, and as stated previously, DEATH.

Types of Illegal/Street Drugs

- ✓ Methamphetamine
- ✓ Opium
- ✓ Bath salts
- ✓ Ecstasy
- ✓ LSD
- ✓ Cocaine
- ✓ Heroin
- ✓ Rohypnol

Stress and Anxiety

I am sure you have heard these words a thousand times, STRESS, and ANXIETY.

When I was having palpitations, and I would go to the ER, I always heard anxiety. I wanted to shake them and say "I DON'T HAVE ANXIETY", "I HAVE PALPITATIONS". I know that for you it may not be anxiety as well; however, someone who reads this book may be suffering from anxiety.

Stress and anxiety is a part of life. No matter who you are, one time or another you have experienced stress and anxiety. Maybe, you have lost your job, a bad breakup, or some other tragic event in your life, like palpitations. Everyone handles stress different, but we all have stress.

Stress can take a toll on the body. A person who is experiencing a lot of stress in their life may contribute stress to them having an ulcer, high blood pressure, or colitis. With that being said, stress can contribute to heart conditions such as a heart attack, chest pains, and palpitations. Stress does not cause the condition per se; however, stress can trigger the condition to cause an onset.

Therefore, it is important for you to manage your stress. Find ways to avoid stress in your life. Remove yourself from stressful situations. Talk with someone. Relax; take a long walk in the park. Try taking a long car drive, a hot bath, or give yoga a try.

Remember stress can onset anxiety; however, other factors can also cause anxiety such as worrying. In some cases, anxiety can literally interrupt your entire life in more ways than one. Anxiety can send your heart beating out of your chest. Furthermore, anxiety can lead to panic attacks. Panic attacks can cause shortness of breath and cause the heart to beat fast.

Another form of anxiety is social anxiety. Social anxiety can cause an increase in heart rate and or hyperventilation when the person is around others. Also, phobia is another form of anxiety. When a person is afraid of something such as spiders then the person may experience various symptoms such as palpitations under frightening situations.

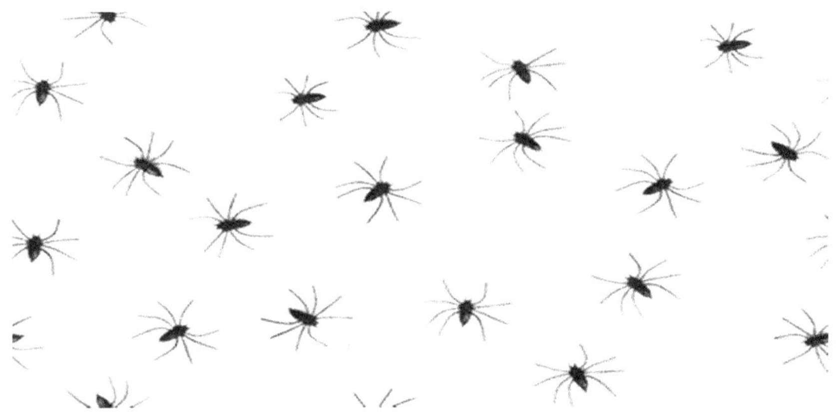

CONCLUSION

This book was designed as a quick reference to help guide you into finding relief from arrhythmia. I cut through all the filler words to get straight to the point. As I stated earlier, I have suffered from palpitations and did find relief. I researched, googled, and asked questions, just like you. That is why I wrote this book. I compiled all the reputable solutions I could find that have worked for me and people just like you.

During my fight with palpitations, I was turned away from my cardiologist and physician and told I would have to live with palpitations the rest of my life. I was told different ways to manage my palpitations, such as relax, breath in your nose, out my mouth, and cut out the anxiety in my life.

No one had the real answer.

Therefore, I had to research this subject myself, only to find that millions of people all around the world have been living with palpitations for years. I had to find relief for us all. Fortunately, I suffered from a hormonal imbalance and found relief from my palpitations by using HRT and incorporating a combination of magnesium and calcium; however, a relative of mine found relief with just aloe juice. We both have since been palpitation free.

There is hope and there is a relief for your palpitations! You know your body, your symptoms, and your trigger signs better than anyone. Use this book to find relief for your symptoms. Don't give up!

You got this!

I wish you luck! I know how your quality of life has changed drastically.

References

1) 6 Health Benefits of Aloe Vera Juice for Your Heart (2018) https://universityhealthnews.com/daily/heart-health/6-health-benefits-of-aloe-vera-juice-for-your-heart/

2) Agatston, A. (2018) The Link Between Magnesium and Heart. Retrieved April 1, 2018 from Health https://www.everydayhealth.com/heart-health-specialist/magnesium.aspx

3) Aloe vera and Heart palpitations - from FDA reports (2018) Retrieved April 1, 2018 from https://www.ehealthme.com/ds/aloe-vera/heart-palpitations/

4) Brisson, J. (2016) Can Stomach Issues Cause Heart Disease? Part 2: Roemheld Syndrome Retrieved March 30, 2018 from https://fixyourgut.com/can-stomach-issues-cause-heart-disease/

5) Caffeine: (2018) How much is too much? https://www.mayoclinic.org/healthy-lifestyle/nutrition-and-healthy-eating/in-depth/caffeine/art-20045678

6) Causes of Heart Palpitations Are Not What You Think (2017) Retrieved April 110, 2018 from https://www.easy-immune-health.com/causes-of-heart-palpitations.html

7) DeNoon, D. (2012) How Much Caffeine Is in Your Energy Drink? https://www.webmd.com/food-recipes/news/20121025/how-much-caffeine-energy-drink#1

8) Felman, A. (2017) Everything you need to know about electrolytes. Retrieved April 10, 2018 from https://www.medicalnewstoday.com/articles/153188.php

9) Fletcher, J., (2017) POTS syndrome: Symptoms, causes, and treatment
https://www.medicalnewstoday.com/articles/320098.php

10) Gastric bug link to irregular heart rhythm, atrial fibrillation (2005). Retrieved April 9, 2018 from https://www.medicalnewstoday.com/releases/26239.php#

11) Laskowski, E. (2018) What's a normal resting heart rate? Retrieved April 16, 2018 from https://www.mayoclinic.org/healthy-lifestyle/fitness/expert-answers/heart-rate/faq-20057979

12) Magnesium in diet (2016) Retrieves April 8, 2018 from https://medlineplus.gov/ency/article/002423.htm

13) Michos, E. (n.d.) Vitamin D and the Heart. Retrieved April 10, 2018 from https://www.hopkinsmedicine.org/heart_vascular_institute/clinical_services/centers_excellence/womens_cardiovascular_health_center/patient_information/health_topics/vitamin_d_and_the_heart.html

14) National Institute of Health Office of Dietary Supplement (2018) https://ods.od.nih.gov/factsheets/Magnesium-HealthProfessional/

15) Sanjay, G., (2015, July 20). Heart palpitations: Proof that magnesium works for ectopic heart beats [Video File]. Retrieved April 10, 2018 from http://www.spring.org.uk/the1sttranspor

16) Zeratsky, K (2018) What is MSG? Is it bad for you? https://www.mayoclinic.org/healthy-lifestyle/nutrition-and-healthy-eating/expert-answers/monosodium-glutamate/faq-20058196